My Pain Recovery Journal

My PAIN RECOVERY *Journal*

"First, believe there is another way to live."

A Day without Pain

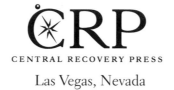

CENTRAL RECOVERY PRESS

Las Vegas, Nevada

CENTRAL RECOVERY PRESS

Central Recovery Press (CRP) is committed to publishing exceptional materials addressing addiction treatment, recovery, and behavioral health care, including original and quality books, audio/visual communications, and web-based new media. Through a diverse selection of titles, it seeks to impact the behavioral health care field with a broad range of unique resources for professionals, recovering individuals, and their families, and the general public. For more information, visit www.centralrecoverypress.com.

Central Recovery Press, Las Vegas, NV 89129
© 2011 by Central Recovery Press, Las Vegas, NV

ISBN-13: 978-0-9799869-7-0
ISBN-10: 0-9799869-7-4

17 16 15 14 13 12 11   1 2 3 4 5

Publisher: Central Recovery Press
             3371 N. Buffalo Drive
             Las Vegas, NV 89129

Cover design and interior by Sara Streifel, Think Creative Design

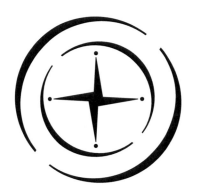

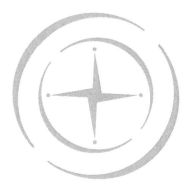

Introduction

Pain is a troublesome companion on our journey toward recovery and is usually looked at as "the enemy." Pain is also referred to as the touchstone of growth. Let's face it, we cannot live our lives without some amount of pain and suffering. In fact, the Buddha told us about this 2500 years ago in his Four Noble Truths.

This journal is meant to be a place to reflect on your responses to pain on a daily basis with an eye toward reducing your suffering. You will see that the more you resist the pain, the more pain you experience (physical and emotional).

It is important to understand that all pain is real, whether it is physical or emotional. Pain develops in the central nervous system and is different in different people. If your pain has become the primary focus of your life, it is time to change. The solutions you will find by journaling daily will include insights about your pain and how you resist it, get angry at it, tighten up in response to it, and become depressed and frustrated with it. All of this makes your pain worse.

Use this journal as a resource. Just putting your thoughts down on paper slows the process down so you can examine it in a mindful and balanced fashion. I have found by working with pain (my own and that of my patients), I am able to diminish suffering. It is paradoxical and will not seem natural, at first, to relax and breathe when you are hurting. With time and consistent effort, you will get used to it and derive the benefits of such a practice. This journal will help you examine your thoughts, emotions, and actions with a detached eye. The more you recognize these processes, the more you will be able to change them, and consequently reduce your pain and suffering.

I wish you well on the journey.

Mel Pohl, MD, FASAM

Author of A Day without Pain and co-author of Pain Recovery: How to Find Balance and Reduce Suffering from Chronic Pain and Pain Recovery for Families: How to Find Balance When Someone Else's Chronic Pain Becomes Your Problem Too

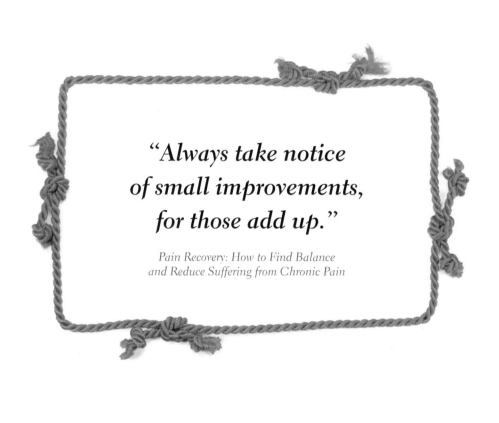

> "Always take notice
> of small improvements,
> for those add up."
>
> *Pain Recovery: How to Find Balance
> and Reduce Suffering from Chronic Pain*

TODAY'S DATE _____

A GOAL FOR TODAY _____

I consider my pain to be _____

_____

_____

_____

_____

_____

_____

_____

_____

Today I realized my pain was less when _____

_____

_____

_____

_____

_____

_____

_____

_____

TODAY'S DATE _____

A GOAL FOR TODAY _____

My greatest fear has been _____

_____

_____

_____

_____

_____

_____

_____

_____

Today I will deal with my fear by _____

_____

_____

_____

_____

_____

_____

_____

_____

TODAY'S DATE _____

A GOAL FOR TODAY _____

I am hopeful about _____

_____

_____

_____

_____

_____

_____

_____

_____

_____

It's been a long time since I _____

_____

_____

_____

_____

_____

_____

_____

_____

TODAY'S DATE _____

A GOAL FOR TODAY _____

I'm practicing _____

_____

_____

_____

_____

_____

_____

_____

I'm really good at _____

_____

_____

_____

_____

_____

_____

_____

_____

TODAY'S DATE _____

A GOAL FOR TODAY _____

When I am hurting I _____

_____

_____

_____

_____

_____

_____

_____

_____

One small step I can take to feel better physically is _____

_____

_____

_____

_____

_____

_____

_____

TODAY'S DATE _____

A GOAL FOR TODAY _____

I think more clearly when I _____

_____

_____

_____

_____

_____

One small step I can take to feel better mentally is _____

_____

_____

_____

_____

_____

"You can detach from your thoughts: observe them,
question their accuracy, dispute or talk back to them,
and ultimately, change them."

Pain Recovery: How to Find Balance and Reduce Suffering from Chronic Pain

TODAY'S DATE _____

A GOAL FOR TODAY _____

Right now I feel _____

_____

_____

_____

_____

_____

_____

_____

_____

One small step I can take to feel better emotionally is _____

_____

_____

_____

_____

_____

_____

_____

_____

TODAY'S DATE _____

A GOAL FOR TODAY _____

The most important things in my life are _____

_____

_____

_____

_____

_____

_____

_____

One small step I can take to feel better spiritually is _____

_____

_____

_____

_____

_____

_____

_____

TODAY'S DATE _____

A GOAL FOR TODAY _____

Health means _____

_____

_____

_____

_____

_____

_____

_____

What I want from my pain recovery program is _____

_____

_____

_____

_____

_____

_____

_____

TODAY'S DATE _____

A GOAL FOR TODAY _____

One positive thought I had today was _____

_____

_____

_____

_____

_____

_____

_____

_____

One positive action I took today was _____

_____

_____

_____

_____

_____

_____

_____

_____

TODAY'S DATE _____

A GOAL FOR TODAY _____

My worst day was _____

_____

_____

_____

_____

_____

To get out of self-pity I _____

_____

_____

_____

_____

_____

_____

> *"Focus on all you are able to do,*
> *rather than dwelling on the things you can no longer do."*
>
> A Day without Pain

TODAY'S DATE _____

A GOAL FOR TODAY _____

My best day was _____

_____

_____

_____

_____

_____

_____

_____

I believe I can _____

_____

_____

_____

_____

_____

_____

_____

TODAY'S DATE _____

A GOAL FOR TODAY _____

I am sorry that I never _____

_____

_____

_____

_____

_____

_____

_____

Before my chronic pain, I _____

_____

_____

_____

_____

_____

_____

_____

TODAY'S DATE _____

A GOAL FOR TODAY _____

I understand powerlessness to mean _____

_____

_____

_____

_____

_____

_____

_____

I feel empowered when I _____

_____

_____

_____

_____

_____

_____

_____

TODAY'S DATE _____

A GOAL FOR TODAY _____

I think a lot about _____

_____

_____

_____

_____

_____

_____

_____

I stop replaying old tapes of "I can't" by _____

_____

_____

_____

_____

_____

_____

_____

TODAY'S DATE _____

A GOAL FOR TODAY _____

At this moment acceptance means _____

_____

_____

_____

_____

_____

I accept that _____

_____

_____

_____

_____

_____

_____

> *"Acceptance is about being okay with situations
> and other people as they are, rather than focusing on
> how I may want them to be or believe they should be."*
>
> *Tails of Recovery: Addicts and the Pets That Love Them*

TODAY'S DATE _____

A GOAL FOR TODAY _____

There are some things no one can take from me, such as _____

_____

_____

_____

_____

_____

_____

_____

_____

Just for today I will _____

_____

_____

_____

_____

_____

_____

_____

_____

TODAY'S DATE _____

A GOAL FOR TODAY _____

When I look in the mirror I see _____

_____

_____

_____

_____

_____

_____

_____

_____

I am making amends to myself by _____

_____

_____

_____

_____

_____

_____

_____

_____

TODAY'S DATE _____

A GOAL FOR TODAY _____

I'm glad I'm able to enjoy _____

_____

_____

_____

_____

_____

_____

_____

Today I'll help someone else by _____

_____

_____

_____

_____

_____

_____

_____

_____

TODAY'S DATE _____

A GOAL FOR TODAY _____

Pain recovery is _____

_____

_____

_____

_____

_____

_____

_____

The most important lesson I have learned in pain recovery thus far is _____

_____

_____

_____

_____

_____

_____

_____

TODAY'S DATE _____

A GOAL FOR TODAY _____

I used to think pain meant _____

_____

_____

_____

_____

_____

Today I will deal with my pain by _____

_____

_____

_____

_____

_____

_____

"Challenge the assumptions you have about your pain."

Pain Recovery: How to Find Balance and Reduce Suffering from Chronic Pain

TODAY'S DATE _____

A GOAL FOR TODAY _____

I am angry about _____

_____

_____

_____

_____

_____

_____

_____

I have learned to cope with my anger by _____

_____

_____

_____

_____

_____

_____

_____

_____

TODAY'S DATE _____

A GOAL FOR TODAY _____

When I need support I _____

_____

_____

_____

_____

_____

_____

_____

_____

I give back by _____

_____

_____

_____

_____

_____

_____

_____

_____

TODAY'S DATE _____

A GOAL FOR TODAY _____

When I hear certain songs, I feel happy; songs like _____

_____

_____

_____

_____

_____

_____

_____

_____

Today I want to _____

_____

_____

_____

_____

_____

_____

_____

_____

TODAY'S DATE _____

A GOAL FOR TODAY _____

I sleep better at night when _____

_____

_____

_____

_____

_____

_____

_____

Each day I will _____

_____

_____

_____

_____

_____

_____

_____

_____

TODAY'S DATE _____

A GOAL FOR TODAY _____

When I suffer I _____

_____

_____

_____

_____

_____

My functioning improves when I _____

_____

_____

_____

_____

_____

*"The suffering that accompanies chronic pain
(your emotional responses) is often much greater
than the pain itself."*

Pain Recovery: How to Find Balance and Reduce Suffering from Chronic Pain

TODAY'S DATE _____

A GOAL FOR TODAY _____

I reached out today and called _____

_____

_____

_____

_____

_____

_____

_____

_____

The best advice I have received thus far is _____

_____

_____

_____

_____

_____

_____

_____

_____

TODAY'S DATE _____

A GOAL FOR TODAY _____

I feel anxious about _____

_____

_____

_____

_____

_____

_____

_____

To alleviate my anxiety I will _____

_____

_____

_____

_____

_____

_____

_____

TODAY'S DATE _____

A GOAL FOR TODAY _____

I feel better physically when I _____

_____

_____

_____

_____

_____

_____

_____

I feel better mentally when I _____

_____

_____

_____

_____

_____

_____

_____

_____

TODAY'S DATE _____

A GOAL FOR TODAY _____

I feel better emotionally when I _____

_____

_____

_____

_____

_____

_____

I feel better spiritually when I _____

_____

_____

_____

_____

_____

_____

_____

TODAY'S DATE _____

A GOAL FOR TODAY _____

I am grateful that I can _____

_____

_____

_____

_____

_____

My experience of pain has taught me _____

_____

_____

_____

_____

_____

_____

> *"With an attitude of gratitude, life's 'problems' can be seen for what they offer—opportunities for growth."*
>
> Recovery A to Z: A Handbook of Twelve-Step Key Terms and Phrases

TODAY'S DATE _____

A GOAL FOR TODAY _____

My highest priority is _____

_____

_____

_____

_____

_____

_____

_____

After my first year in pain recovery I want to _____

_____

_____

_____

_____

_____

_____

_____

TODAY'S DATE _____

A GOAL FOR TODAY _____

Today surrender means _____

_____

_____

_____

_____

_____

_____

_____

_____

When I feel afraid I _____

_____

_____

_____

_____

_____

_____

_____

_____

TODAY'S DATE _____

A GOAL FOR TODAY _____

Something I cannot change is _____

_____

_____

_____

_____

_____

_____

_____

_____

Something I can change is _____

_____

_____

_____

_____

_____

_____

_____

_____

TODAY'S DATE _____

A GOAL FOR TODAY _____

Beautiful colors remind me that _____

_____

_____

_____

_____

_____

_____

_____

Today I will deal with my sadness by _____

_____

_____

_____

_____

_____

_____

_____

TODAY'S DATE _____

A GOAL FOR TODAY _____

Pain isn't the only thing in my life; there's also _____

_____

_____

_____

_____

_____

Today I will deal with my frustration by _____

_____

_____

_____

_____

_____

_____

> *"The pain you feel is not you;*
> *it is simply the pain you feel."*
>
> A Day without Pain

TODAY'S DATE _____

A GOAL FOR TODAY _____

I describe myself as _____

_____

_____

_____

_____

_____

_____

_____

_____

I felt good about myself today when _____

_____

_____

_____

_____

_____

_____

_____

_____

TODAY'S DATE _____

A GOAL FOR TODAY _____

I look forward to _____

_____

_____

_____

_____

_____

_____

_____

Wisdom I can use today is _____

_____

_____

_____

_____

_____

_____

_____

TODAY'S DATE _____

A GOAL FOR TODAY _____

To connect with others I _____

_____

_____

_____

_____

_____

_____

_____

_____

To connect with my higher power I _____

_____

_____

_____

_____

_____

_____

_____

_____

TODAY'S DATE _____

A GOAL FOR TODAY _____

Today I'm focused on _____

_____

_____

_____

_____

_____

_____

_____

To help me relax I _____

_____

_____

_____

_____

_____

_____

_____

TODAY'S DATE _____

A GOAL FOR TODAY _____

Mindfulness means _____

_____

_____

_____

_____

_____

When I meditate I _____

_____

_____

_____

_____

_____

_____

"Meditation can encourage a sense of well-being,
happiness, connectedness, and wholeness."

A Day without Pain

TODAY'S DATE _____

A GOAL FOR TODAY _____

I wish I could _____

_____

_____

_____

_____

_____

_____

_____

_____

I have made a choice to _____

_____

_____

_____

_____

_____

_____

_____

_____

TODAY'S DATE _____

A GOAL FOR TODAY _____

I am learning to cope with my pain by _____

_____

_____

_____

_____

_____

_____

_____

I've noticed an improvement in _____

_____

_____

_____

_____

_____

_____

_____

TODAY'S DATE _____

A GOAL FOR TODAY _____

I get strength from _____

_____

_____

_____

_____

_____

_____

_____

My purpose is _____

_____

_____

_____

_____

_____

_____

_____

TODAY'S DATE _____

A GOAL FOR TODAY _____

Today my pain differs from my first day in pain recovery because _____

_____

_____

_____

_____

_____

_____

_____

Hope means _____

_____

_____

_____

_____

_____

_____

_____

_____

TODAY'S DATE _____

A GOAL FOR TODAY _____

Commitment means _____

_____

_____

_____

_____

_____

I stay committed to my recovery by _____

_____

_____

_____

_____

_____

"Commitment is undoubtedly one of the cornerstones
of a solid recovery program."

Tails of Recovery: Addicts and the Pets That Love Them

TODAY'S DATE _____

A GOAL FOR TODAY _____

When I feel angry about my pain, in order to better accept it I _____

_____

_____

_____

_____

_____

_____

_____

I can change how I think about my pain by _____

_____

_____

_____

_____

_____

_____

_____

_____

TODAY'S DATE _____

A GOAL FOR TODAY _____

Everything I do doesn't have to be perfect; it can be good enough. I am

a good enough _____

_____

_____

_____

_____

_____

_____

When I feel low, I treat myself to _____

_____

_____

_____

_____

_____

_____

_____

TODAY'S DATE _____

A GOAL FOR TODAY _____

I counteract self-pity by _____

_____

_____

_____

_____

_____

_____

_____

_____

I remain conscious of everything I have to be grateful for by _____

_____

_____

_____

_____

_____

_____

_____

_____

TODAY'S DATE _____

A GOAL FOR TODAY _____

When others "just don't understand," I find it beneficial to _____

_____

_____

_____

_____

_____

_____

_____

Others have taught me that _____

_____

_____

_____

_____

_____

_____

_____

TODAY'S DATE _____

A GOAL FOR TODAY _____

When I feel lonely, I _____

_____

_____

_____

_____

_____

I can receive support from _____

_____

_____

_____

_____

_____

_____

"Being able to receive [support] requires admitting there are some things you can't and shouldn't attempt to do on your own."

Pain Recovery: How to Find Balance and Reduce Suffering from Chronic Pain

TODAY'S DATE _____

A GOAL FOR TODAY _____

In meditation today I _____

_____

_____

_____

_____

_____

_____

_____

_____

Today I will take the time to _____

_____

_____

_____

_____

_____

_____

_____

_____

TODAY'S DATE _____

A GOAL FOR TODAY _____

I'm still me, even with my pain. One of the best things about me is _____

_____

_____

_____

_____

_____

_____

_____

I am inspired by _____

_____

_____

_____

_____

_____

_____

_____

TODAY'S DATE _____

A GOAL FOR TODAY _____

I maintain awareness that how I feel is different from how I choose to act by

_____

_____

_____

_____

_____

_____

_____

_____

I take comfort in _____

_____

_____

_____

_____

_____

_____

_____

TODAY'S DATE _____

A GOAL FOR TODAY _____

When my recovery seems to reach a plateau, I _____

_____

_____

_____

_____

_____

_____

_____

When fear starts to creep into my awareness, it is helpful for me to _____

_____

_____

_____

_____

_____

_____

_____

TODAY'S DATE _____

A GOAL FOR TODAY _____

When family and friends react negatively to my situation, I _____

_____

_____

_____

_____

_____

To feel more connected to my loved ones, I _____

_____

_____

_____

_____

_____

_____

*"Let go of your sense of being 'different' and
any fear you may have of other people criticizing you."*

A Day without Pain

TODAY'S DATE _____

A GOAL FOR TODAY _____

Today I'll wear my favorite shirt/hat/sweater. I love it because _____

_____

_____

_____

_____

_____

_____

_____

One thing that always makes me happy is _____

_____

_____

_____

_____

_____

_____

_____

TODAY'S DATE _____

A GOAL FOR TODAY _____

When my negative thinking is getting the best of me, I _____

_____

_____

_____

_____

_____

_____

_____

When I begin to blame others for the way I feel, I remind myself that _____

_____

_____

_____

_____

_____

_____

_____

TODAY'S DATE _____

A GOAL FOR TODAY _____

I am reaching out by _____

_____

_____

_____

_____

_____

_____

_____

One thing I will do for myself today is _____

_____

_____

_____

_____

_____

_____

_____

_____

TODAY'S DATE _____

A GOAL FOR TODAY _____

I've learned that _____

_____

_____

_____

_____

_____

_____

_____

_____

I am still struggling with _____

_____

_____

_____

_____

_____

_____

_____

_____

TODAY'S DATE _____

A GOAL FOR TODAY _____

Today "showing up" means _____

_____

_____

_____

_____

_____

I am learning to trust that _____

_____

_____

_____

_____

_____

"Being trusting lets us simplify our lives by showing up, doing the best we can, and then relaxing and enjoying whatever happens."

Of Character: Building Assets in Recovery

TODAY'S DATE _____

A GOAL FOR TODAY _____

I feel more peaceful when _____

_____

_____

_____

_____

_____

_____

_____

To develop my spirituality, I _____

_____

_____

_____

_____

_____

_____

_____

TODAY'S DATE _____

A GOAL FOR TODAY _____

Last night I felt _____

_____

_____

_____

_____

_____

_____

_____

Now I am feeling _____

_____

_____

_____

_____

_____

_____

_____

_____

TODAY'S DATE _____

A GOAL FOR TODAY _____

To maintain an awareness of my emotions, I _____

_____

_____

_____

_____

_____

_____

_____

_____

When I am having a difficult day, I will remember _____

_____

_____

_____

_____

_____

_____

_____

_____

TODAY'S DATE _____

A GOAL FOR TODAY _____

I have _____

_____

_____

_____

_____

_____

_____

_____

_____

I am _____

_____

_____

_____

_____

_____

_____

_____

_____

TODAY'S DATE _____

A GOAL FOR TODAY _____

I can tell I am engaging in faulty thinking when _____

_____

_____

_____

_____

_____

To restore balanced thoughts I _____

_____

_____

_____

_____

_____

*"Sometimes our faults can lead us, through suffering,
to do good; so no one need feel ashamed."*

Recovery A to Z: A Handbook of Twelve-Step Key Terms and Phrases

TODAY'S DATE _____

A GOAL FOR TODAY _____

Today I will be mindful of _____

_____

_____

_____

_____

_____

_____

_____

I "get out of myself" by _____

_____

_____

_____

_____

_____

_____

_____

_____

TODAY'S DATE _____

A GOAL FOR TODAY _____

My favorite therapy is _____

_____

_____

_____

_____

_____

_____

_____

This therapy helps me by _____

_____

_____

_____

_____

_____

_____

_____

TODAY'S DATE _____

A GOAL FOR TODAY _____

I intend to _____

_____

_____

_____

_____

_____

_____

_____

My higher power _____

_____

_____

_____

_____

_____

_____

_____

_____

TODAY'S DATE _____

A GOAL FOR TODAY _____

I believe that _____

_____

_____

_____

_____

_____

_____

_____

_____

Today serenity means _____

_____

_____

_____

_____

_____

_____

_____

_____

TODAY'S DATE _____

A GOAL FOR TODAY _____

My pain has made me realize _____

_____

_____

_____

_____

_____

One thing I am sure of is _____

_____

_____

_____

_____

_____

*"The power of our beliefs
can transcend physical conditions."*

A Day without Pain

TODAY'S DATE _____

A GOAL FOR TODAY _____

Every day I am committed to _____

_____

_____

_____

_____

_____

_____

_____

A life goal of mine is _____

_____

_____

_____

_____

_____

_____

_____

TODAY'S DATE _____

A GOAL FOR TODAY _____

I am having difficulty with _____

_____

_____

_____

_____

_____

_____

_____

When I am tempted to medicate with something, instead I _____

_____

_____

_____

_____

_____

_____

_____

TODAY'S DATE _____

A GOAL FOR TODAY _____

I feel _____

_____

_____

_____

_____

_____

_____

_____

_____

In order to give myself permission to feel whatever I am feeling, I _____

_____

_____

_____

_____

_____

_____

_____

_____

TODAY'S DATE _____

A GOAL FOR TODAY _____

To stay in the present moment I _____

_____

_____

_____

_____

_____

_____

_____

_____

Right now I _____

_____

_____

_____

_____

_____

_____

_____

_____

TODAY'S DATE _____

A GOAL FOR TODAY _____

I deal with feelings of grief and loss by _____

_____

_____

_____

_____

_____

To avoid isolating myself I _____

_____

_____

_____

_____

_____

_____

"Without question, feeling grief and accepting the reality of loss are two of the biggest challenges in recovery."

Tails of Recovery: Addicts and the Pets That Love Them

TODAY'S DATE _____

A GOAL FOR TODAY _____

Something that made me happy today was _____

_____

_____

_____

_____

_____

_____

_____

_____

My favorite book, movie, song is _____ because

_____

_____

_____

_____

_____

_____

_____

_____

TODAY'S DATE _____

A GOAL FOR TODAY _____

Today I improved my conscious contact with my higher power by_____

_____

_____

_____

_____

_____

_____

_____

_____

Just for today I will do one selfless act of _____

_____

_____

_____

_____

_____

_____

_____

_____

TODAY'S DATE _____

A GOAL FOR TODAY _____

I understand helplessness to mean _____

_____

_____

_____

_____

_____

_____

_____

I am proud of myself for _____

_____

_____

_____

_____

_____

_____

_____

_____

TODAY'S DATE _____

A GOAL FOR TODAY _____

Today I will deal with any anxiety, fear, or pain by _____

_____

_____

_____

_____

_____

_____

_____

To lower my stress level I _____

_____

_____

_____

_____

_____

_____

_____

TODAY'S DATE _____

A GOAL FOR TODAY _____

I am able to _____

_____

_____

_____

_____

_____

Something I've always wanted to do is _____

_____

_____

_____

_____

_____

_____

"You are powerless over your pain and the circumstances that created it. However, you are not helpless."

A Day without Pain

TODAY'S DATE _____

A GOAL FOR TODAY _____

I know I can always talk to _____

_____

_____

_____

_____

_____

_____

_____

One thing I have done to improve my communication skills is _____

_____

_____

_____

_____

_____

_____

_____

_____

TODAY'S DATE _____

A GOAL FOR TODAY _____

I am willing to _____

_____

_____

_____

_____

_____

_____

_____

I am hopeful about _____

_____

_____

_____

_____

_____

_____

_____

_____

TODAY'S DATE _____

A GOAL FOR TODAY _____

I am dealing with my resentments by _____

_____

_____

_____

_____

_____

_____

_____

_____

I practice being more patient by _____

_____

_____

_____

_____

_____

_____

_____

TODAY'S DATE _____

A GOAL FOR TODAY _____

I've come to understand _____

_____

_____

_____

_____

_____

_____

_____

I feel positive about _____

_____

_____

_____

_____

_____

_____

_____

TODAY'S DATE _____

A GOAL FOR TODAY _____

Today I feel _____

_____

_____

_____

_____

_____

When I find myself resisting my pain, I _____

_____

_____

_____

_____

_____

"The more you attempt to avoid, mask, and medicate,
the greater your suffering will be."

Pain Recovery: How to Find Balance and Reduce Suffering from Chronic Pain

TODAY'S DATE _____

A GOAL FOR TODAY _____

Just for today I believe I can _____

_____

_____

_____

_____

_____

_____

_____

I need _____

_____

_____

_____

_____

_____

_____

_____

TODAY'S DATE _____

A GOAL FOR TODAY _____

Today I want to _____

_____

_____

_____

_____

_____

_____

_____

My pain is _____

_____

_____

_____

_____

_____

_____

_____

TODAY'S DATE _____

A GOAL FOR TODAY _____

Some things I am doing to take better care of my health are _____

_____

_____

_____

_____

_____

_____

_____

I am learning to be more gentle with myself by _____

_____

_____

_____

_____

_____

_____

_____

TODAY'S DATE _____

A GOAL FOR TODAY _____

When I think about my pain I feel _____

_____

_____

_____

_____

_____

_____

_____

When I am engaging in victim-thinking I _____

_____

_____

_____

_____

_____

_____

_____

TODAY'S DATE _____

A GOAL FOR TODAY _____

I never thought I would _____

_____

_____

_____

_____

_____

I now understand _____

_____

_____

_____

_____

_____

_____

*"Recovery necessitates the ability
to accept life on its own terms."*

Tails of Recovery: Addicts and the Pets That Love Them

TODAY'S DATE _____

A GOAL FOR TODAY _____

I treat myself well by _____

_____

_____

_____

_____

_____

_____

_____

I treat others well by _____

_____

_____

_____

_____

_____

_____

_____

TODAY'S DATE _____

A GOAL FOR TODAY _____

Today I am grateful for _____

_____

_____

_____

_____

_____

_____

_____

Some things that help me feel more balanced are _____

_____

_____

_____

_____

_____

_____

_____

_____

TODAY'S DATE _____

A GOAL FOR TODAY _____

When I am feeling discouraged I will _____

_____

_____

_____

_____

_____

_____

_____

I feel stronger when I _____

_____

_____

_____

_____

_____

_____

_____

TODAY'S DATE _____

A GOAL FOR TODAY _____

In spite of my pain, I _____

_____

_____

_____

_____

_____

_____

_____

It encourages me when _____

_____

_____

_____

_____

_____

_____

_____

_____

TODAY'S DATE _____

A GOAL FOR TODAY _____

I find meaning in my experience by _____

_____

_____

_____

_____

_____

My pain has taught me _____

_____

_____

_____

_____

_____

_____

*"Accept your pain and cherish the opportunities
it provides you to grow and change."*

Pain Recovery: How to Find Balance and Reduce Suffering from Chronic Pain

TODAY'S DATE _____

A GOAL FOR TODAY _____

I keep a positive outlook by _____

_____

_____

_____

_____

_____

_____

_____

The last time I felt joy, I was _____

_____

_____

_____

_____

_____

_____

_____

_____

TODAY'S DATE _____

A GOAL FOR TODAY _____

Some changes in my physical self have been _____

_____

_____

_____

_____

_____

_____

_____

I nourish my body by _____

_____

_____

_____

_____

_____

_____

_____

_____

TODAY'S DATE _____

A GOAL FOR TODAY _____

The changes that have been the hardest to adjust to are _____

_____

_____

_____

_____

_____

_____

_____

I am learning to accept these changes by _____

_____

_____

_____

_____

_____

_____

_____

TODAY'S DATE _____

A GOAL FOR TODAY _____

My best attributes are _____

_____

_____

_____

_____

_____

_____

_____

I always feel better when I _____

_____

_____

_____

_____

_____

_____

_____

TODAY'S DATE _____

A GOAL FOR TODAY _____

Lately I have been worrying about _____

_____

_____

_____

_____

_____

To deal with my worries and fears I _____

_____

_____

_____

_____

_____

_____

> *"When we acknowledge and face our fears,*
> *energy is freed for other spiritual pursuits."*
>
> *Of Character: Building Assets in Recovery*

TODAY'S DATE _____

A GOAL FOR TODAY _____

I feed my spirituality by _____

_____

_____

_____

_____

_____

_____

_____

One thing that has helped my healing is _____

_____

_____

_____

_____

_____

_____

_____

TODAY'S DATE _____

A GOAL FOR TODAY _____

Intuition means _____

_____

_____

_____

_____

_____

_____

_____

I listen to my inner voice by _____

_____

_____

_____

_____

_____

_____

_____

_____

TODAY'S DATE _____

A GOAL FOR TODAY _____

One thing that is holding me back right now is _____

_____

_____

_____

_____

_____

_____

_____

One thing that will help me move forward is _____

_____

_____

_____

_____

_____

_____

_____

TODAY'S DATE _____

A GOAL FOR TODAY _____

When I feel resistant to receiving help and support, I overcome it by _____

_____

_____

_____

_____

_____

_____

_____

_____

I share my experience, strength, and hope by _____

_____

_____

_____

_____

_____

_____

_____

_____

TODAY'S DATE _____

A GOAL FOR TODAY _____

Giving makes me feel _____

_____

_____

_____

_____

_____

Receiving makes me feel _____

_____

_____

_____

_____

_____

_____

*"Seek and accept support from family, friends, therapists,
and support groups. You don't have to do this alone."*

A Day without Pain

TODAY'S DATE _____

A GOAL FOR TODAY _____

I know that _____

_____

_____

_____

_____

_____

_____

_____

I deal with fear of the unknown by _____

_____

_____

_____

_____

_____

_____

_____

TODAY'S DATE _____

A GOAL FOR TODAY _____

My faith is strengthened by _____

_____

_____

_____

_____

_____

_____

_____

_____

What matters most to me is _____

_____

_____

_____

_____

_____

_____

_____

_____

TODAY'S DATE _____

A GOAL FOR TODAY _____

One thing I see differently now is _____

_____

_____

_____

_____

_____

_____

_____

Some thoughts and beliefs I have had about my pain that I am now

challenging are _____

_____

_____

_____

_____

_____

_____

TODAY'S DATE _____

A GOAL FOR TODAY _____

I strongly believe that _____

_____

_____

_____

_____

_____

_____

_____

_____

I am still trying to figure out _____

_____

_____

_____

_____

_____

_____

_____

_____

TODAY'S DATE _____

A GOAL FOR TODAY _____

I find the strength to get through a difficult day by _____

_____

_____

_____

_____

_____

I feel closest to my higher power when _____

_____

_____

_____

_____

_____

_____

*"Faith, hope, and trust are fundamental components
of the pain-recovery process."*

Pain Recovery: How to Find Balance and Reduce Suffering from Chronic Pain

TODAY'S DATE _____

A GOAL FOR TODAY _____

I give myself permission to _____

_____

_____

_____

_____

_____

_____

_____

Today I will ask for help with _____

_____

_____

_____

_____

_____

_____

_____

TODAY'S DATE _____

A GOAL FOR TODAY _____

I am capable of _____

_____

_____

_____

_____

_____

_____

_____

_____

A new skill I would like to learn is _____

_____

_____

_____

_____

_____

_____

_____

TODAY'S DATE _____

A GOAL FOR TODAY _____

I have made a lot of progress with _____

_____

_____

_____

_____

_____

_____

_____

_____

I'm practicing _____

_____

_____

_____

_____

_____

_____

_____

_____

TODAY'S DATE _____

A GOAL FOR TODAY _____

I am adapting to _____

_____

_____

_____

_____

_____

_____

_____

Accepting where I am today helps me _____

_____

_____

_____

_____

_____

_____

_____

_____

TODAY'S DATE _____

A GOAL FOR TODAY _____

When I find myself asking "why me?" I _____

_____

_____   _____

_____

_____

_____

I deal with the unfairness of chronic pain by _____

_____

_____

_____

_____

_____

_____

"Recognizing that you are angry, depressed, or stressed out because of your pain may mean you can exert some control over the level of pain affecting you."

A Day without Pain

TODAY'S DATE _____

A GOAL FOR TODAY _____

Physically I feel _____

_____

_____

_____

_____

_____

_____

_____

My "daily maintenance" routine for my body includes _____

_____

_____

_____

_____

_____

_____

_____

TODAY'S DATE _____

A GOAL FOR TODAY _____

Mentally I am _____

_____

_____

_____

_____

_____

_____

_____

Each day I work on my state of mind by _____

_____

_____

_____

_____

_____

_____

_____

TODAY'S DATE _____

A GOAL FOR TODAY _____

Emotionally I feel _____

_____

_____

_____

_____

_____

_____

_____

I practice awareness of my feelings by _____

_____

_____

_____

_____

_____

_____

_____

TODAY'S DATE _____

A GOAL FOR TODAY _____

My spiritual health is _____

_____

_____

_____

_____

_____

_____

_____

I stay spiritually connected by _____

_____

_____

_____

_____

_____

_____

_____

_____

TODAY'S DATE _____

A GOAL FOR TODAY _____

When I am angry, the feelings that are usually behind it are _____

_____

_____

_____

_____

_____

Identifying these feelings helps me deal with my anger by _____

_____

_____

_____

_____

_____

_____

*"Feelings are nothing to fear, although it may feel as if
they are to be feared when they first emerge."*

Recovery A to Z: A Handbook of Twelve-Step Key Terms and Phrases

TODAY'S DATE _____

A GOAL FOR TODAY _____

I need to remind myself to _____

_____

_____

_____

_____

_____

_____

_____

I feel good about _____

_____

_____

_____

_____

_____

_____

_____

_____

TODAY'S DATE _____

A GOAL FOR TODAY _____

I have started to notice _____

_____

_____

_____

_____

_____

_____

_____

_____

I have changed my mind about _____

_____

_____

_____

_____

_____

_____

_____

TODAY'S DATE _____

A GOAL FOR TODAY _____

When I reflect on the past year, I think _____

_____

_____

_____

_____

_____

_____

_____

_____

I feel _____

_____

_____

_____

_____

_____

_____

_____

_____

TODAY'S DATE _____

A GOAL FOR TODAY _____

I feel hopeful when _____

_____

_____

_____

_____

_____

_____

_____

_____

Just for today I will _____

_____

_____

_____

_____

_____

_____

_____

_____

TODAY'S DATE _____

A GOAL FOR TODAY _____

I am being of service to others by _____

_____

_____

_____

_____

_____

When I give back I _____

_____

_____

_____

_____

_____

_____

*"When we are presented with the opportunity to be generous,
our first reaction should be one of gratitude that we
have anything worthwhile to give, followed by awareness
that whatever we share we get to keep."*

Of Character: Building Assets in Recovery

TODAY'S DATE _____

A GOAL FOR TODAY _____

My pain is _____

_____

_____

_____

_____

_____

_____

_____

One area of imbalance I am working on is _____

_____

_____

_____

_____

_____

_____

_____

_____

TODAY'S DATE _____

A GOAL FOR TODAY _____

I dream about _____

_____

_____

_____

_____

_____

_____

_____

_____

One dream that has come true is _____

_____

_____

_____

_____

_____

_____

_____

_____

TODAY'S DATE _____

A GOAL FOR TODAY _____

I practiced honesty today by _____

_____

_____

_____

_____

_____

_____

_____

One way my work has paid off is _____

_____

_____

_____

_____

_____

_____

_____

TODAY'S DATE _____

A GOAL FOR TODAY _____

This week I accomplished _____

_____

_____

_____

_____

_____

_____

_____

What keeps me motivated is _____

_____

_____

_____

_____

_____

_____

_____

TODAY'S DATE _____

A GOAL FOR TODAY _____

I feel out of balance when _____

_____

_____

_____

_____

_____

When I am having "one of those days," I make sure to _____

_____

_____

_____

_____

_____

_____

"Balance is not static but fluid, in a constant state of flux, much like the ebb and flow of the waves on the ocean."

Pain Recovery: How to Find Balance and Reduce Suffering from Chronic Pain

TODAY'S DATE _____

A GOAL FOR TODAY _____

I feel balanced when _____

_____

_____

_____

_____

_____

_____

_____

_____

One thing I do to restore my balance is _____

_____

_____

_____

_____

_____

_____

_____

_____

TODAY'S DATE _____

A GOAL FOR TODAY _____

In this moment I _____

_____

_____

_____

_____

_____

_____

_____

I feel a sense of purpose when I _____

_____

_____

_____

_____

_____

_____

_____

TODAY'S DATE _____

A GOAL FOR TODAY _____

I laughed today when _____

_____

_____

_____

_____

_____

_____

_____

I always have fun when I _____

_____

_____

_____

_____

_____

_____

_____

_____

TODAY'S DATE _____

A GOAL FOR TODAY _____

I would like to be able to _____

_____

_____

_____

_____

_____

_____

_____

There are things I can do today that I couldn't do yesterday, like _____

_____

_____

_____

_____

_____

_____

_____

TODAY'S DATE _____

A GOAL FOR TODAY _____

I am optimistic about _____

_____

_____

_____

_____

When I become aware of negative thoughts I _____

_____

_____

_____

_____

_____

"Being willing to acknowledge and accept your emotions and feel them as they arise may help remove their negative power."

A Day without Pain

TODAY'S DATE _____

A GOAL FOR TODAY _____

Things that I have or do that contribute to my identity include _____

_____

_____

_____

_____

_____

_____

_____

_____

These things are important to my sense of self because _____

_____

_____

_____

_____

_____

_____

_____

_____

TODAY'S DATE _____

A GOAL FOR TODAY _____

Some positive qualities I've identified in my character are _____

_____

_____

_____

_____

_____

_____

_____

Some negative qualities I've identified in my character are _____

_____

_____

_____

_____

_____

_____

_____

TODAY'S DATE _____

A GOAL FOR TODAY _____

Some messages I received about pain during childhood include _____

_____

_____

_____

_____

_____

_____

_____

One memory I have of a painful experience is _____

_____

_____

_____

_____

_____

_____

_____

TODAY'S DATE _____

A GOAL FOR TODAY _____

My stress level is usually _____

_____

_____

_____

_____

_____

_____

_____

One thing that relaxes me is _____

_____

_____

_____

_____

_____

_____

_____

_____

TODAY'S DATE _____

A GOAL FOR TODAY _____

My physical reactions to stress are _____

_____

_____

_____

_____

_____

I relax my body by _____

_____

_____

_____

_____

_____

"Frustration and anger lead to increased muscle tension and stress, which generally lead to increased sensations of pain."

Pain Recovery: How to Find Balance and Reduce Suffering from Chronic Pain

TODAY'S DATE _____

A GOAL FOR TODAY _____

My mental reactions to stress are _____

_____

_____

_____

_____

_____

_____

_____

I calm my mind by _____

_____

_____

_____

_____

_____

_____

_____

TODAY'S DATE _____

A GOAL FOR TODAY _____

My emotional reactions to stress are _____

_____

_____

_____

_____

_____

_____

_____

I soothe my feelings by _____

_____

_____

_____

_____

_____

_____

_____

TODAY'S DATE _____

A GOAL FOR TODAY _____

My spiritual reactions to stress are _____

_____

_____

_____

_____

_____

_____

_____

I reconnect with my spirit by _____

_____

_____

_____

_____

_____

_____

_____

_____

TODAY'S DATE _____

A GOAL FOR TODAY _____

My biggest challenge right now is _____

_____

_____

_____

_____

_____

_____

_____

_____

I am succeeding at _____

_____

_____

_____

_____

_____

_____

_____

_____

TODAY'S DATE _____

A GOAL FOR TODAY _____

I work on my patience by _____

_____

_____

_____

_____

_____

I feel calm when _____

_____

_____

_____

_____

_____

"*Being calm gives us the ability to sit with our feelings,
whether those feelings are joyous or painful, and know
we are more than what we feel at that moment.
Being calm helps us remember we are guided and protected.*"

Of Character: Building Assets in Recovery

TODAY'S DATE _____

A GOAL FOR TODAY _____

Lately my pain has been _____

_____

_____

_____

_____

_____

_____

_____

_____

Today I feel _____

_____

_____

_____

_____

_____

_____

_____

_____

TODAY'S DATE _____

A GOAL FOR TODAY _____

Some thoughts I've had today include _____

_____

_____

_____

_____

_____

_____

_____

_____

My emotional responses to these thoughts were _____

_____

_____

_____

_____

_____

_____

_____

TODAY'S DATE _____

A GOAL FOR TODAY _____

My pain seems to increase when _____

_____

_____

_____

_____

_____

_____

_____

My pain seems to decrease when _____

_____

_____

_____

_____

_____

_____

_____

TODAY'S DATE _____

A GOAL FOR TODAY _____

When I'm having a bad pain day, I _____

_____

_____

_____

_____

_____

_____

_____

I am determined to _____

_____

_____

_____

_____

_____

_____

_____

_____

TODAY'S DATE _____

A GOAL FOR TODAY _____

I feel more in control when _____

_____

_____

_____

_____

_____

I deal with things I cannot control by _____

_____

_____

_____

_____

_____

*"Identifying the things you cannot change, as well as what
you can do to better accept those things, will make noticeable,
positive differences in your experience of pain and in your life."*

Pain Recovery: How to Find Balance and Reduce Suffering from Chronic Pain

TODAY'S DATE _____

A GOAL FOR TODAY _____

Some obstacles that might affect my pain recovery are _____

_____

_____

_____

_____

_____

_____

_____

My solutions to these obstacles are _____

_____

_____

_____

_____

_____

_____

_____

TODAY'S DATE _____

A GOAL FOR TODAY _____

Some thoughts I've had today include _____

_____

_____

_____

_____

_____

_____

_____

My emotional responses to these thoughts were _____

_____

_____

_____

_____

_____

_____

_____

TODAY'S DATE _____

A GOAL FOR TODAY _____

I believe in my ability to _____

_____

_____

_____

_____

_____

_____

_____

The steps I will take to reach my goal for today are _____

_____

_____

_____

_____

_____

_____

_____

_____

TODAY'S DATE _____

A GOAL FOR TODAY _____

When I feel powerless I _____

_____

_____

_____

_____

_____

_____

_____

No one can make me _____

_____

_____

_____

_____

_____

_____

_____

_____

TODAY'S DATE _____

A GOAL FOR TODAY _____

I express my creativity in pain recovery by _____

_____

_____

_____

_____

_____

My vision for the future includes _____

_____

_____

_____

_____

_____

*"Creativity in recovery allows us…to see a number
of possible solutions to a problem then select
the one that creates the best possible outcome."*

Of Character: Building Assets in Recovery

TODAY'S DATE _____

A GOAL FOR TODAY _____

Writing in this journal is helping me to_____

_____

_____

_____

_____

_____

_____

_____

_____

The best advice I've received lately is _____

_____

_____

_____

_____

_____

_____

_____

TODAY'S DATE _____

A GOAL FOR TODAY _____

I stay actively involved in pain recovery by _____

_____

_____

_____

_____

_____

_____

_____

Today my functioning is _____

_____

_____

_____

_____

_____

_____

_____

TODAY'S DATE _____

A GOAL FOR TODAY _____

One thing I would like to do differently is _____

_____

_____

_____

_____

_____

_____

_____

My perspective has changed about _____

_____

_____

_____

_____

_____

_____

_____

TODAY'S DATE _____

A GOAL FOR TODAY _____

When I was a kid I always wanted _____

_____

_____

_____

_____

_____

_____

_____

My life would be different if I'd never met _____

_____

_____

_____

_____

_____

_____

_____

_____

TODAY'S DATE _____

A GOAL FOR TODAY _____

I am learning to let go of _____

_____

_____

_____

_____

_____

I stay in the present by _____

_____

_____

_____

_____

_____

*"Happiness, joy, and serenity
are only possible in the present."*

Recovery A to Z: A Handbook of Twelve-Step Key Terms and Phrases

TODAY'S DATE _____

A GOAL FOR TODAY _____

The "gift" of my experience with chronic pain has been _____

_____

_____

_____

_____

_____

_____

_____

Today balance means _____

_____

_____

_____

_____

_____

_____

_____

_____

TODAY'S DATE _____

A GOAL FOR TODAY _____

One place in the world I really want to go is _____

_____

_____

_____

_____

_____

_____

_____

I used to think _____

_____

_____

_____

_____

_____

_____

_____

_____

TODAY'S DATE _____

A GOAL FOR TODAY _____

One thing I can do today for my health is _____

_____

_____

_____

_____

_____

_____

_____

One feeling I'm having right now is _____

_____

_____

_____

_____

_____

_____

_____

_____

TODAY'S DATE _____

A GOAL FOR TODAY _____

This week I will call _____

_____

_____

_____

_____

_____

_____

_____

This week I will visit _____

_____

_____

_____

_____

_____

_____

_____

TODAY'S DATE _____

A GOAL FOR TODAY _____

I miss _____

_____

_____

_____

_____

_____

I am working through my grief about _____

_____

_____

_____

_____

_____

"When you experience significant loss—whether by death, divorce, illness, or other circumstance—give yourself the gift of feeling grief, whatever form it may take and however long it lasts."

The Soul Workout: Getting and Staying Spiritually Fit

TODAY'S DATE _____

A GOAL FOR TODAY _____

My biggest fear is _____

_____

_____

_____

_____

_____

_____

_____

Today "living in the solution" means _____

_____

_____

_____

_____

_____

_____

_____

TODAY'S DATE _____

A GOAL FOR TODAY _____

Today I am grateful for _____

_____

_____

_____

_____

_____

_____

_____

I express my gratitude by _____

_____

_____

_____

_____

_____

_____

_____

TODAY'S DATE _____

A GOAL FOR TODAY _____

My experience with resentments is _____

_____

_____

_____

_____

_____

_____

_____

_____

I forgive _____

_____

_____

_____

_____

_____

_____

_____

_____

My Pain Recovery Journal

TODAY'S DATE _____

A GOAL FOR TODAY _____

I remember a time when I _____

_____

_____

_____

_____

_____

_____

_____

One thing that has changed is _____

_____

_____

_____

_____

_____

_____

_____

_____

TODAY'S DATE _____

A GOAL FOR TODAY _____

To me, change is _____

_____

_____

_____

_____

_____

I'm ready to _____

_____

_____

_____

_____

_____

_____

"Identify something that you know you need to change
about yourself. Are you ready to make that change?
If yes, what do you need to do to start? If no, what needs
to happen in order for you to be ready?"

The Soul Workout: Getting and Staying Spiritually Fit

TODAY'S DATE _____

A GOAL FOR TODAY _____

The last time I felt sad was because _____

_____

_____

_____

_____

_____

_____

_____

Today I know _____

_____

_____

_____

_____

_____

_____

_____

_____

TODAY'S DATE _____

A GOAL FOR TODAY _____

For me, "a good life" means _____

_____

_____

_____

_____

_____

_____

_____

When I feel like my needs aren't being met, I _____

_____

_____

_____

_____

_____

_____

_____

TODAY'S DATE _____

A GOAL FOR TODAY _____

The best advice I can give to others with chronic pain is _____

_____

_____

_____

_____

_____

_____

_____

_____

Today I shared with others by _____

_____

_____

_____

_____

_____

_____

_____

TODAY'S DATE _____

A GOAL FOR TODAY _____

When I need support I can reach out to _____

_____

_____

_____

_____

_____

_____

_____

I show my appreciation for my support system by _____

_____

_____

_____

_____

_____

_____

_____

_____

TODAY'S DATE _____

A GOAL FOR TODAY _____

My pain has taught me _____

_____

_____

_____

_____

_____

Today I define my progress in pain recovery as _____

_____

_____

_____

_____

_____

_____

"If we are grateful for the opportunity to recover and live based on spiritual principles, then we know that everything, even pain, offers a gift or gifts."

Of Character: Building Assets in Recovery

TODAY'S DATE _____

A GOAL FOR TODAY _____

My favorite activity to take my mind off my pain is _____

_____

_____

_____

_____

_____

_____

_____

If I could spend today doing anything, I would _____

_____

_____

_____

_____

_____

_____

_____

TODAY'S DATE _____

A GOAL FOR TODAY _____

When I feel frustrated with my doctor/provider I _____

_____

_____

_____

_____

_____

_____

_____

I consider it a good day when _____

_____

_____

_____

_____

_____

_____

_____

_____

TODAY'S DATE _____

A GOAL FOR TODAY _____

Dear Chronic Pain _____

_____

_____

_____

_____

_____

_____

_____

_____

Today I feel _____

_____

_____

_____

_____

_____

_____

_____

TODAY'S DATE _____

A GOAL FOR TODAY _____

The last thing I cried about was _____

_____

_____

_____

_____

_____

Today I define my progress in pain recovery as _____

_____

_____

_____

_____

_____

_____

> *"The harder I tried to be powerful and overcome the pain, the more powerless and in pain I was. The more I resisted, the worse I hurt."*
>
> *A Day without Pain*

TODAY'S DATE _____

A GOAL FOR TODAY _____

When I don't feel motivated to do what my doctor/provider tells me to, I _____

_____

_____

_____

_____

_____

_____

_____

I am taking care of myself today by _____

_____

_____

_____

_____

_____

_____

_____

TODAY'S DATE _____

A GOAL FOR TODAY _____

My pain today is _____

_____

_____

_____

_____

_____

_____

_____

My emotional state right now can best be described as _____

_____

_____

_____

_____

_____

_____

_____

TODAY'S DATE _____

A GOAL FOR TODAY _____

Balance means _____

_____

_____

_____

_____

_____

_____

_____

_____

What I most want others to understand about me is _____

_____

_____

_____

_____

_____

_____

_____

TODAY'S DATE _____

A GOAL FOR TODAY _____

I retrospect, I wish I hadn't _____

_____

_____

_____

_____

_____

_____

_____

I am glad I _____

_____

_____

_____

_____

_____

_____

_____

_____

TODAY'S DATE _____

A GOAL FOR TODAY _____

When I'm feeling sorry for myself I find it helpful to _____

_____

_____

_____

_____

_____

_____

_____

_____

I maintain a good attitude by _____

_____

_____

_____

_____

_____

_____

_____

_____

TODAY'S DATE _____

A GOAL FOR TODAY _____

To me, acceptance means _____

_____

_____

_____

_____

_____

I am working on accepting _____

_____

_____

_____

_____

_____

_____

"When we are accepting in recovery, we 'receive' others, the world, our circumstances, and ourselves 'as adequate.' This does not mean we must be content with things exactly as they are. It means we learn to align ourselves with and acknowledge reality."

Of Character: Building Assets in Recovery

TODAY'S DATE _____

A GOAL FOR TODAY _____

I feel loved when _____

_____

_____

_____

_____

_____

_____

_____

A valuable lesson I have learned is _____

_____

_____

_____

_____

_____

_____

_____

TODAY'S DATE _____

A GOAL FOR TODAY _____

I have come to believe that _____

_____

_____

_____

_____

_____

_____

_____

_____

Something that is challenging me right now is _____

_____

_____

_____

_____

_____

_____

_____

TODAY'S DATE _____

A GOAL FOR TODAY _____

Pain recovery has helped me grow in these ways _____

_____

_____

_____

_____

_____

_____

_____

_____

A good day is when _____

_____

_____

_____

_____

_____

_____

_____

TODAY'S DATE _____

A GOAL FOR TODAY _____

My highest priority is _____

_____

_____

_____

_____

_____

_____

_____

Pain recovery has made me truly appreciate _____

_____

_____

_____

_____

_____

_____

_____

TODAY'S DATE _____

A GOAL FOR TODAY _____

My experience with expectations has been _____

_____

_____

_____

_____

_____

When others aren't meeting my needs, _____

_____

_____

_____

_____

_____

_____

"Whenever you think in terms of how people or situations should be, you set yourself up for disappointment."

Pain Recovery: How to Find Balance and Reduce Suffering from Chronic Pain

TODAY'S DATE _____

A GOAL FOR TODAY _____

Some of my automatic thoughts are _____

_____

_____

_____

_____

_____

_____

_____

I am working on positive thinking by _____

_____

_____

_____

_____

_____

_____

_____

TODAY'S DATE _____

A GOAL FOR TODAY _____

Rather than avoiding certain situations or feelings, I_____

_____

_____

_____

_____

_____

_____

_____

I have made peace with _____

_____

_____

_____

_____

_____

_____

_____

_____

TODAY'S DATE _____

A GOAL FOR TODAY _____

I am powerless over _____

_____

_____

_____

_____

_____

_____

_____

I work on my need for control by _____

_____

_____

_____

_____

_____

_____

_____

_____

_____

TODAY'S DATE _____

A GOAL FOR TODAY _____

My journey with pain is _____

_____

_____

_____

_____

_____

_____

_____

When I become consumed with negative or worrisome thoughts, I will _____

_____

_____

_____

_____

_____

_____

_____

TODAY'S DATE _____

A GOAL FOR TODAY _____

I share my experience, strength, and hope by _____

_____

_____

_____

_____

_____

Just for today I _____

_____

_____

_____

_____

_____

_____

*"The more you learn, the more you will be able
to help someone else who is in pain with encouragement
and information about your experience."*

A Day without Pain